Sugar Detox Diet For Beginners:

Lose Weight, Increase Your Energy and Look Younger

By

Brittany Samons

Table of Contents

Introduction 5

Chapter 1. Main Principles of Sugar Detox Diet 6

Chapter 2. Sugar Detox Diet and Weight Loss 8

Chapter 3. Sugar Detox Diet and Energy 9

Chapter 4. How Sugar Detox Diet Makes You Younger 10

Chapter 5. Foods to Eat and Foods to Avoid 11

Chapter 6. Food Plan 14

    Meal Plan 1 15

    Meal Plan 2 16

Chapter 7. Sugar Detox Diet Recipes 18

    1. Breakfast Recipes 18

    2. Lunch and Dinner Recipes 22

    3. Snack Recipes 25

Final Words 27

Thank You Page 29

Sugar Detox Diet For Beginners: Lose Weight, Increase Your Energy and Look Younger

By Brittany Samons

© Copyright 2014 Brittany Samons

Reproduction or translation of any part of this work beyond that permitted by section 107 or 108 of the 1976 United States Copyright Act without permission of the copyright owner is unlawful. Requests for permission or further information should be addressed to the author.

This publication is designed to provide accurate and authoritative information in regard to the subject matter covered. This work is sold with the understanding that the publisher is not engaged in rendering legal, accounting, or other professional services. If legal advice or other expert assistance is required, the services of a competent professional person should be sought.

First Published, 2014

Printed in the United States of America

Introduction

The sugar detox diet is a new diet plan that is all about reducing, if not totally removing all foods that contain sugar. This diet is based on latest studies that sugar is found to be one of the major causes of various medical problems and not just diabetes. Sugar and not fat is responsible for weight gain and of course all the illnesses that stem from being overweight or obese: from hypertension, cardiac diseases and depression. Sugar is also the leading cause of skin disorders like acne and pimples, dementia and reproductive disorders like infertility and impotence.

And it seems that it is not that easy to get rid of sugar in our daily diets. Aside from foods that we know are loaded with sugar, it is hard to spot foods that contain hidden sugar. Almost all processed foods and manufactured foods are loaded with flavors and preservatives that are composed of sugars. Junk foods and commercially –prepared beverages also contain high amounts of hidden sugar and thus must be reduced or totally eliminated from the diet to efficiently take advantage of the benefits of this diet.

This book will help you to lower sugar consumption and become healthier.

Chapter 1. Main Principles of Sugar Detox Diet

Sugar detox diet is all about using a diet plan that is contains minimal amounts of sugar to totally removing sugar from all the meals that you take each day. Detoxifying the body from sugar is the purpose of a sugar detox and just like diets that cleanse the body, there are some important things that a sugar detox diet user should remember when starting this diet plan.

First, an average American consumes about 152 pounds of sugar annually; if you put it into a clearer amount, you are consuming about 22 teaspoons of sugar in a day. You may have thought that this is impossible since you hardly use sugar in your coffee and beverages however this much sugar is usually from other foods and drinks that you consume. Therefore you are unaware that your body is taking hidden sugar.

Consuming this much sugar in a day has made more teens suffer from pre-diabetic symptoms while adults as early as their 30s are suffering from diabetes symptoms. Diabetes is a disease that is the underlying cause of so many other health conditions such as hypertension, allergies, kidney disease, skin conditions, glaucoma and so many more. Therefore adapting a low sugar to a sugar detox diet should start as early as possible.

And possibly what only a few people know about sugar is that it is more addicting than cocaine. Therefore sugar addiction is real. Hormones secreted by the body and various neurotransmitters make the body crave for sugar and sugar cravings lead to overeating and eventually obesity. By indulging in a detox diet, the body will be able to counter the effects of sugar addiction and stop dependence to sugar for good.

Chapter 2. Sugar Detox Diet and Weight Loss

A sugar detox diet is able to help anyone that would like to lose weight because it stops the cycle of sugar addiction. Detoxifying the body is getting rid of the substance that is causing harm and in the case of sugar detox training; you are getting rid of sugar to reduce its hazardous effects.

Obesity is the result of continuous intake of sugar. Remember that the body naturally loves sugar and the more you take in sugar the more your body becomes addictive to it and the end result is becoming overweight or obese. By interrupting the cycle of sugar addiction and by using exercise and a complete lifestyle change, you will be able to gradually lose weight. Maintaining an ideal weight may be done through the use of a sugar-free diet and to switching to a healthy lifestyle that totally avoids the intake of sugar.

Chapter 3. Sugar Detox Diet and Energy

As you begin to use the sugar detox diet you will eventually experience a period when your blood sugar levels are stable. At this period you are more able to do a variety of physical activities since you have an increased amount of energy to spare. You are able to walk for longer period of hours without the familiar fatigue plus you may already engage in more strenuous activities like exercise. Your thyroid glands also benefits from stable sugar levels; your thyroid functions return to normal and this helps you feel more active and able to withstand longer and more strenuous physical activities.

Chapter 4. How Sugar Detox Diet Makes You Younger

As you are able to withstand exercise and physical activities you will be able to improve your physical appearance in the long run. You will feel energized and revitalized with this increase in energy since when you exercise and do all sorts of physical activity you increase blood supply to the different body systems. Your heart beats faster and thus all the body systems benefit.

Your skin looks smoother, healthier and glossier since there is increase in blood supply to the organ. Your hair looks shinier and full of volume due to an increase in blood supply to the scalp. You are able to digest your food better and benefit from the nutrients and energy that you get from food since there is also improved blood supply to the gastrointestinal system. You feel alert, able to concentrate and able to make quick decisions when there is increased blood supply to the brain. All in all, your body feels younger and better after getting rid of sugar addiction that has been causing damage to your body systems.

Chapter 5. Foods to Eat and Foods to Avoid

In a sugar detox diet you need to remove all foods that contain sugar as well as foods that are made from flour. You may eat all the rest of the foods that do not contain sugar and flour. It may sound easy but actually it may be quite challenging since when you check out food labels you can always find these ingredients listed. Other foods may not even have an adequate list of ingredients that will warn you of sugar and flour content. Beverages also have high levels of sugar especially carbonated sodas, energy drinks and commercially prepared juices therefore these should be totally avoided. All in all, you must avoid the following foods: alcohol, artificial sweeteners, breads, candy, breakfast cereals, dairy products, flour tortillas, canned or packaged fruit juices, potatoes, corn syrup, honey, maple syrup, oatmeal, cane sugar, sucrose, trans fats, wheat breads and pasta, white breads and flour, rice and yoghurt.

It is important to note that artificial sweeteners are on the list. Artificial sweeteners only fuel your sugar addiction more since you still cling on using sugar and you still crave sugar in your foods. Going cold turkey may be the only answer to finally getting rid of a sugar addiction.

When it comes to the foods that you can eat, there are a lot to choose from. Sugar is the foundation of our body's energy stores and you may have thought that sugar from carbohydrates that you eat is the only way that the body can fuel itself each day. However, a better source of energy is protein. Protein can help balance blood sugar and insulin through stopping your sugar cravings. Therefore in the list of foods that you can eat, you will find a lot of protein-rich food sources. Foods that you can indulge in when you are in a sugar detox diet are herbs, all kinds of vegetables, avocadoes, beans, brown rice, eggs, fish, lentils, nuts, olive oil, free-range chicken, turkey, beef and lamb, seeds, tomatoes, salmon and yams.

All protein sources like chicken, turkey, beef and lamb should be organic since these have the highest quality protein. Fish should be bought fresh as well as all vegetables should be eaten fresh too. Eating fresh and organic food ensures that the body is getting adequate amounts of protein that is needed for energy in a sugar detox diet.

But of course aside from learning the foods that you must avoid and which foods you may eat is just the first part of doing a sugar detox diet. You should also prepare these foods using a sugar-free method. For instance you should cook fish, poultry and meats in a manner that preserves its nutrients and still promotes sugar detox; a good way to do this is by broiling or steaming food since it cooks in its own flavor and no additional ingredients are added that may have hidden sugars. Broiling and grilling are another great ways to prepare food but easy on using sauces like barbeque sauce, marinara sauces or soy sauce that may also contain sugar. You are detoxifying your body from sugar and it may be useless to avoid foods that contain sugar when you are secretly taking it in.

Chapter 6. Food Plan

A sugar detox diet is achieved with the use of a comprehensive meal plan that covers what you eat from breakfast till dinner time. A typical detox diet lasts for five to ten days depending on the program that you are in. there are numerous sugar detox diet that you may see on the web but all in all these diet plans focus on eliminating sugar and flour. And although these diets may take on different names, the end result is still the same, all focus on the benefits that the body gets from detoxifying from sugar: weight loss, better health, more energy and a younger and lighter feeling.

The best way to come up with a food plan is to first look at the foods list that you may eat and choose the foods that you would like to have for breakfast, lunch, dinner and snacks. You must also base your diet according to the number of calories that you need in a day. A sugar detox diet does not restrict the number of calories that you take in each day but since the foods that have the highest amounts of calories are foods that are loaded with sugar and flour then you may need to develop a meal plan that will contain enough calories to sustain your needs in a day.

Meal Plan 1

Breakfast

Ham and organic cheese omelet

An apple

Freshly-squeezed juice

Lunch

Braised short ribs

Taco salad

Dinner

Baked chicken thighs

Grilled asparagus

Fruit cups for dessert

Snacks

Bacon, lettuce and tomato sandwich

Meal Plan 2

Breakfast

Almond flour pancakes

A piece of melon

Lunch

Garlic ginger chicken

Avocado and olive salad

½ cup of brown rice

Dinner

Spicy cinnamon lamb steak

Green beans

Snacks

Tacos in Jicama shells

It is best to avoid consuming any food after 8 in the evening especially when you do not have any other activities planned during these hours. Your body consumes only a few calories digesting food and snacking will only contribute to weight gain. If you are used to eating a snack before a meal then you may feel uneasy and hungry during the first few days of your diet plan but experts reveal that feeling hunger during these hours may only signal that you are thirsty or dehydrated. Drinking water may help reduce hunger pangs in the evening.

Foods that are found in these two meal plans are prepared with ingredients that are free from sugar and any kind of flour. Each meal is composed of foods that are found in the what to eat list and are also cooked without added sugar and flour. Understanding how to cook meals following a sugar detox diet plan is easy when you use sugar detox diet recipes.

Chapter 7. Sugar Detox Diet Recipes

1. Breakfast Recipes

Bacon, Beef and Eggs High Protein Breakfast Treat

As mentioned, you will need a lot of proteins to improve your energy levels and this breakfast treat gives you the protein that you need to fuel your energy. You will need 4 big pieces of bacon, 1 medium-sized green onion, sliced, a cup of green cabbage, shredded, a teaspoon of organic coconut oil, a dash of salt and pepper and 3 pasteurized eggs.

Prepare your oven by heating it to 500 degrees Fahrenheit. Use a medium sized baking sheet and then place the bacon pieces on the sheet, set this aside. Use a medium-sized frying pan and heat a teaspoon of coconut oil in medium heat. Place the green cabbage and then sauté until cooked, add the dash of salt and pepper and remove from heat. Fry eggs in a pan using the remaining oil and then when eggs are cooked set these aside with the cooked cabbage. Place the bacon in the oven and then broil. You may need to flip the bacon once or twice to ensure that it cooked through. Serve together in a plate right after the bacon is cooked.

Breakfast Frittata

This dish is a wonderful combination of veggies and meat that will fill you with energy during breakfast and will keep you full till lunch. No need to eat a snack plus you will also find the vitamins and minerals that you need for the day. You need a cup of spinach, a cup of white mushrooms, a tablespoon of coconut oil, 3 pieces of asparagus, ¾ cup of yellow onion, 8 whole eggs, a teaspoon of black pepper and salt.

Prepare your vegetables by chopping them into small pieces, set them aside. Prepare your oven by heating it to 350 degrees Fahrenheit. Use an oven-safe pan or skillet; heat about ½ tablespoons of coconut oil in medium heat. Cook vegetables for 3 minutes in the pan until the onions are flavorful and translucent in color; the mushrooms should be soft which means these are cooked. Remove from heat once the veggies are cooked. Whish 8 eggs in a medium-sized bowl and then stir in the veggies and mushrooms. Heat another ½ teaspoons of coconut oil in a skillet and then pour the mixture to cook for another 4 to 5 minutes. Place the mixture in the oven and then bake for 10 minutes. You will know that your breakfast frittata is ready when the eggs are spongy in texture. Remove from the oven-safe skillet and then slice. You may place chopped bacon on top of the frittata slices along with chopped green pepper.

Breakfast Muffins Made from Egg

Eggs are a great source of protein and are also very versatile. In this recipe you will be able to cook eggs just like muffins and the best thing about this recipe is you could take your breakfast anywhere. You will need 8 pasteurized eggs, a teaspoon of salt, ½ teaspoon of coconut oil, a cup of broccoli, ½ cup broccoli, ½ onion, ¼ green bell peppers, ¼ red bell peppers and a dash of pepper.

Prepare your oven to 400 degrees Fahrenheit. Use a muffin tin and prepare it by greasing it lightly with coconut oil. Chop all the vegetables into very small pieces. When your veggies are ready, divide them according to the number of muffin tins. Whisk all the eggs in a large bowl land then pour these into the muffin tins with vegetables. Add salt and pepper in each tin; stir with a teaspoon to distribute the vegetables in the egg. Place the muffin tin in the oven and then bake for 20 minutes. The egg muffins are ready when the top part of the muffin is soft and spongy. Place a few pieces of chopped vegetables and ground pepper on top just before you serve.

Vanilla Flavored Pancakes

Instead of using plain flour you will find that using coconut flour is easier; you may never even be able to tell any changes in flavor and taste too. You will need ¼ baking soda, ¼ cup of coconut flour, a dash of salt, 4 medium pasteurized eggs, a tablespoon of vanilla extract and a tablespoon of water.

You will need a handheld mixer or a stand up mixer to blend all the ingredients in a large mixing bowl: blend the eggs, water, salt, baking soda and vanilla. As the mixture is blending, pour the coconut flour part by part into the bowl. Continue doing so until all the flour has been added to the mixture. Continue to blend until you have achieved a smooth mixture. Use a non-stick pan to cook the pancakes. Heat a tablespoon of butter (organic and grass-fed) over medium heat. With the use of a soup ladle, pour the mixture gently over the butter and then cook. Flip the pancakes accordingly and then allow each side to cook for at least a minute before turning. If the pancake still looks soft and runny, continue to cook by flipping it for another minute more. Serve with butter (organic and grass-fed) or with fruits.

2. Lunch and Dinner Recipes

Lamb Roast

This is a slow cook recipe to make the lamb roast tender and more flavorful. You can have this on a special weekend for lunch or dinner. You will need a rack of lamb or about 2 pounds of lamb chops, a cup of water, a sprig of rosemary, a teaspoon of salt, a head of garlic, about 10 olives and a dash of black pepper.

Prepare the garlic by separating the cloves, peeling and smashing them. Use a large crock pot to cook your roast; place the roast in a position that will allow the meaty portion of the roast to be exposed to heat. Top the roast with garlic, olive juice, olives, salt and pepper. Place water under the crack pot. Place the herbs on the roast and then cook with the cover on. This recipe should be done ahead of time since you will need to spend at least 8 to 10 hours of cooking time just to achieve a soft and well-cooked rack of lamb. When the roast is ready, divide the rack into small pieces.

Smoked Shrimp with Vegetables

This recipe is made of fresh vegetables and tasty shrimp that is a refreshing change from meat and poultry dishes. You will need a tablespoon of garlic, a teaspoon of smoked paprika, 2 pounds of shrimp, ½ cup of parsley, ½ head of cabbage, ¼ cup of carrot, ¼ cups of green onion, 2/3 cup of celery, 2/3 cup of radish, 2 tablespoons of palm oil, 4 large strips of bacon, a dash of pepper and a dash of salt.

Prepare the vegetables by rinsing and then chopping these into very small pieces. Clean the shrimps and then place these in a large mixing bowl along with the salt, pepper, paprika, oil and minced garlic. Use a large non-stick frying pan to sauté the shrimps until these develop a pink color which means that these are already cooked. Remove the shrimp and set aside when they are done. Cook the bacon strips in medium heat until these are tasty and crispy. Remove these from heat and then cool. Chop into very small pieces. Add the shrimps to the vegetables and then toss. Sprinkle these with chopped bacon and serve.

Mint and Pesto Lamb Meatballs

Lamb meatballs, mint and pesto make a great dish for lunch or dinner. You may need to allot a few minutes to prepare the meatballs or you may do this the evening before and store meatballs in the fridge using an airtight container. You will need a whole pasteurized egg, a teaspoon of salt, a teaspoon of oregano, a teaspoon of garlic powder, a pound of ground lamb, 4 medium-sized zucchinis, a tablespoon of coconut oil, a clove of garlic, a teaspoon of black pepper and 2 tablespoons of mint pesto.

Prepare your oven by heating it to 350 degrees Fahrenheit. Place the ground lamb and all the spices in a large mixing bowl; whisk the egg and then add to the mixture and then mix until all the ingredients are evenly distributed. Use your hands to get a small amount of mixture to form a small ball (the size of golf or a ping pong ball). Place your lamb balls in a baking sheet lined with parchment paper and bake for about 20 to 25 minutes. Chop the zucchinis into small strips then sauté in a skillet in coconut oil, garlic, salt and pepper. Toss in the mint pesto, zucchinis and place the lamb meatballs over the veggies.

3. Snack Recipes

Sugar Detox Fudgy Brownies

This is a recipe that will truly amaze you since these brownies taste pretty much like regular brownies minus the grain. You will need about 5 ounces of dark chocolate, 8 ounces of unsalted butter, a teaspoon of vanilla extract, 4 large-sized eggs, ½ cups of chestnut flour, a dash of sea salt, a teaspoon of baking powder and ¾ cup of coconut sugar.

Preheat your oven to 350 degrees Fahrenheit. Use a baking dish with parchment paper and then grease lightly with unsalted butter. Melt the chocolate in a small skillet on medium heat along with the butter. Be sure to stir continuously. Add the coconut sugar and the vanilla to the mixture and then continue to stir until you have a smooth mixture. Remove from heat and then allow to cool on the counter. In a separate medium-sized bowl blend the eggs, flour, salt and baking powder. Pour the cooled chocolate mixture in and then mix until you achieve a smooth consistency. Pour the batter on the oiled parchment paper. Bake this for about 30 to 40 minutes. Cool the brownies before slicing them into small pieces.

Bacon, Lettuce and Tomato Snack

This is a perfect heavy snack with high quality protein so you will feel energized in the afternoon. You will need a large beefsteak tomato, a teaspoon of garlic powder, a teaspoon of onion powder, a teaspoon of black pepper, a teaspoon of salt, two teaspoons of paprika, a pound of ground bison, 8 large pieces of bacon and 4 pieces of lettuce. You will be able to make about 2 servings with this recipe.

Cook the bacon over medium heat until it is crispy and then set these aside. Heat your grill to medium heat. Combine the ground bison meat, salt, pepper, garlic and paprika powder and onion powder. Mix these until you have a smooth consistency; divide the mixture into four large patties. Grill these burgers until these are completely cooked. You must cook these about 5 minutes per side. Grill the tomatoes as well. Arrange the bacon, patties and the lettuce and then serve.

Final Words

If you may have noticed there are actually only a few differences when it comes to flavor and taste of the meals presented here and in fact you may find that eating sugar detox meals are more flavorful than the usual way you prepare your meals; this is because you are cooking meals using the usual flavor or the ingredients and not relying on synthetic flavors, sugar and other flavors to enhance the taste of the food.

A sugar detox diet is a diet that should last only for a maximum of ten days however you may use this diet plan to completely eliminate sugar and flour from your meals. Remember that you will be able to reap the benefits of indulging in a sugar detox diet only after regular use of the diet. Most people that undergo a sugar detox may feel weak and craving for sugary treats after a day or two but afterwards there are hardly any symptoms of detox from sugar. Some that have successfully used a sugar detox have felt lighter, weighed better and felt healthier which is why most that have used this diet decide to continue it for life. Indulging children to eat sugar free meals is a great idea for parents and caregivers to start especially when there is high incidence of diabetes and weight related problems in children.

Thank You Page

I want to personally thank you for reading my book. I hope you found information in this book useful and I would be very grateful if you could leave your honest review about this book. I certainly want to thank you in advance for doing this.

www.ingramcontent.com/pod-product-compliance
Lightning Source LLC
LaVergne TN
LVHW021748060526
838200LV00052B/3545